THE COMPLETE MIGRAINE DIET COOKBOOK

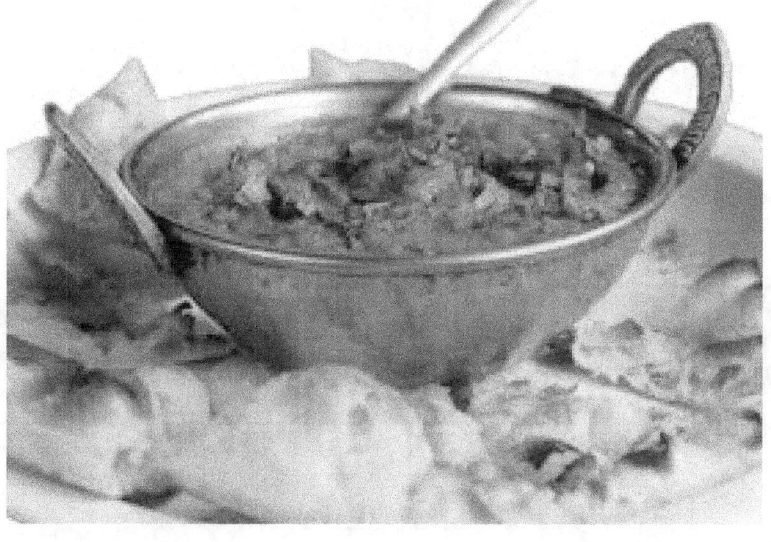

Nourishing Recipes and Comprehensive Meal Plans for Lasting Headache Relief and Optimal Wellness

Isabelle Hartley

OTHER BOOKS BY THIS AUTHOR

1. GASTROPARESIS DIET RECIPES COOKBOOK
2. HIGH CALORIES DIET COOKBOOK
3. DIET FOR WOMEN OVER FORTY
4. HASHIMOTO RECIPES COOKBOOK
5. JUICING RECIPES FOR CANCER
6. IVF DIET COOKBOOK FOR BEGINNERS
7. LOW SUGAR DIET GUIDE FOR BEGINNERS
8. RAW FOODS RECIPES COOKBOOK
9. SMOOTHIES RECIPES FOR ANTI-INFLAMMATION
10. MEDITERRANEAN DIET FOR PREGNANT WOMEN

TABLE OF CONTENTS

Introduction

Allow me to start this book with the story of Rebecca, a 35-year-old working woman who has suffered from frequent migraines for many years. She became dissatisfied with the ongoing discomfort and the several drugs that didn't bring about long-term relief, so she looked into other options. Rebecca set out on a mission to use a specially designed diet to stop her migraines.

Though first dubious, Rebecca conducted a thorough investigation and discovered probable trigger foods that may be causing her migraines. She began by getting rid of usual offenders like coffee, processed meals, and other chemicals. She used full, nutrient-dense meals with anti-inflammatory qualities in lieu of them.

After a few difficult weeks of adjusting to her new diet, Rebecca started to see a noticeable decrease in the frequency and severity of her migraines. Inspired by these initial indications of progress, she persisted in adjusting her diet, concentrating on preserving an equilibrium of vital nutrients.

Rebecca included drinking water into her daily regimen after realizing the importance of staying hydrated in preventing migraines. To determine which meal times and quantity amounts were most effective for her, she tried a variety of approaches. Including frequent, wholesome meals in her diet helped to balance her blood sugar levels, which in turn helped to relieve her migraines.

Months later, Rebecca's success story came to light. She went from being dependent on medications to going weeks at a time without having a single migraine attack. She saw a boost in energy and a greater sense of engagement in her personal and professional lives.

Rebecca's ability to reverse migraines with food changed not just her own life but also the lives of people around her. Her experience demonstrates the significant positive effects on health that can result from eating a balanced, migraine-friendly diet. It is a ray of hope for those who are looking for a long-term, all-natural solution to migraine treatment.

CHAPTER 1

Welcome to "The Migraine Diet Cookbook," a thorough manual created to assist you in using mindful eating to control and maybe even reverse headaches. In these pages, we explore the substantial effects that a well-designed diet may have on relieving the difficulties associated with chronic migraines, and we also look at the transforming power of this approach.

Migraines can greatly lower one's quality of life since they are frequently misdiagnosed and difficult to treat. This cookbook serves as a guide for embracing a lifestyle that prioritizes migraine-friendly eating in addition to being a compilation of recipes. We think that one of the most important factors in your search for healing may be making thoughtful and informed food choices.

We urge you to learn about the principles underlying this methodology in this introductory part. We will go over the fundamentals of migraines, illuminating possible causes and the connection between food and migraine attacks. This information will enable you to choose the foods you eat with understanding, leading to a better and more migraine-resistant life.

Our driving concept is simplicity throughout the cookbook. We understand that changing one's diet may be a big change, so we've made sure that everyone can use our recipes and advice, no matter what level of culinary experience they have. These pages are designed to make your path toward migraine treatment pleasurable and doable, regardless of your level of experience in the kitchen.

Together, let's take this life-changing step and embrace a migraine diet that not only nourishes your body but also has the potential to lead to a life with fewer migraine attacks and an improved quality of life overall.

THE MIGRAINE

Cause, Symptoms And Types

Migraine: Unveiling the Layers of a Complex Condition

Migraine, a neurological disorder characterized by recurring moderate to severe headaches, is much more than a mere headache. The intricate web of causes, diverse symptoms, and various types makes understanding and managing migraines a complex task. In this exploration, we unravel the layers of this condition, shedding light on its causes, symptoms, and the different types that affect millions worldwide.

Causes of Migraine:

The origins of migraines are multifaceted, often involving a combination of genetic, environmental, and lifestyle factors. Genetic predisposition plays a significant role; individuals with a family history of migraines are more likely to experience them.

Alterations in brain activity and imbalances in neurotransmitters, such as serotonin, are implicated in the onset of migraines.

Triggers vary widely among individuals, making it challenging to pinpoint specific causes. Common triggers include certain foods (such as chocolate, aged cheese, and processed meats), hormonal changes (especially in women during menstruation), lack of sleep, stress, environmental factors (like bright lights and strong smells), and changes in weather.

Understanding one's unique set of triggers is crucial for effective migraine management. Keeping a detailed migraine diary can help identify patterns and pinpoint specific triggers, allowing individuals to make informed lifestyle adjustments.

Symptoms of Migraine:

Migraines manifest with a range of symptoms that extend beyond head pain. The classic migraine headache is often described as a pulsating or throbbing pain on one side of the head. However, some individuals may experience pain on both sides or a shifting pain pattern.

Accompanying the headache, various symptoms may manifest in distinct phases:

Prodrome Phase: This phase occurs hours to days before the headache and includes subtle signs like mood swings, food cravings, and increased thirst. Recognizing these early signals can provide a window for preventive measures.

Aura Phase: Not all migraine sufferers experience an aura, but for those who do, it typically involves visual disturbances, such as flashing lights or zigzag lines. Auras can also include sensory changes, such as tingling or numbness in the face or hands.

Headache Phase: This is the most recognizable phase characterized by the throbbing head pain. Accompanying symptoms may include nausea, vomiting, and sensitivity to light and sound.

Postdrome Phase: Following the headache, individuals may experience a postdrome, often described as a "migraine hangover." Fatigue, difficulty concentrating, and lingering head discomfort are common in this phase.

Migraines are highly individualized, and not everyone experiences all phases. The duration and severity of each phase can vary, making each migraine episode a unique experience.

Types of Migraine:

Migraines are classified into several types based on specific characteristics and symptoms. The two main categories are migraine without aura and migraine with aura.

Migraine without Aura: This is the most common type, characterized by moderate to severe pulsating headaches without the preceding aura phase. The headache is often accompanied by nausea, vomiting, and sensitivity to light and sound.

Migraine with Aura: Approximately one-fourth of migraine sufferers experience an aura before the headache. Auras are typically visual disturbances, but they can also involve sensory changes. The aura phase precedes the headache and serves as a warning sign for many individuals.

Beyond these broad categories, migraines can be further classified into subtypes, including chronic migraines (occurring on 15 or more days per month) and vestibular migraines (accompanied by dizziness and balance issues).

In conclusion, migraines are a complex neurological disorder with diverse causes, symptoms, and types. While genetic factors play a role, triggers and individual responses to those triggers vary widely. Recognizing and managing migraines require a personalized approach, involving lifestyle modifications, trigger identification, and, in some cases, medical intervention. As we continue to unravel the mysteries of migraines, a comprehensive understanding of this condition becomes essential for those navigating its challenges and seeking effective management strategies.

What Triggers Migraines

Migraines, often elusive in their exact origins, can be triggered by a variety of factors that vary among individuals. Understanding these triggers is crucial for managing and potentially preventing migraine episodes. Common triggers include:

Food and Beverages: Certain foods and drinks can act as triggers. Common culprits include chocolate, aged cheese, processed meats containing nitrites, caffeine, alcohol, and artificial sweeteners. Identifying and eliminating specific dietary triggers can significantly reduce migraine occurrences.

Hormonal Changes: Fluctuations in hormones, particularly in women, are a well-known trigger. Migraines can be linked to menstrual cycles, pregnancy, and menopause. Hormone-related migraines often occur during the premenstrual phase.

Stress and Emotional Factors: Stress is a significant contributor to migraines. Emotional factors such as anxiety, tension, and even positive excitement can trigger episodes. Developing stress management techniques, like mindfulness and relaxation exercises, is key in mitigating this trigger.

Environmental Factors: Bright lights, loud noises, and strong smells can trigger migraines in susceptible individuals. Changes in weather, especially fluctuations in barometric pressure, can also contribute. Managing exposure to these environmental factors can be beneficial.

Sleep Patterns: Irregular sleep patterns, inadequate sleep, or oversleeping can trigger migraines. Establishing a consistent sleep routine and prioritizing sufficient sleep is crucial for migraine prevention.

Physical Factors: Intense physical activity, especially if not part of a regular routine, can trigger migraines. On the flip side, abrupt cessation of physical activity can also be a trigger. Gradual and consistent exercise, tailored to individual capabilities, is advisable.

Dehydration: Inadequate hydration can lead to migraines. Maintaining a proper fluid balance by drinking enough water throughout the day is a simple yet effective strategy.

Medication Overuse: Ironically, certain medications, if overused, can contribute to migraines. Over-the-counter pain relievers, especially those containing caffeine, can lead to a rebound effect, causing more frequent headaches.

Individuals often experience a combination of these triggers, making it essential to identify patterns through keeping a migraine diary. This personalized approach allows for targeted lifestyle adjustments, empowering individuals to manage and potentially alleviate migraines by avoiding or mitigating specific triggers. By recognizing and addressing these triggers, individuals can take proactive steps towards a more migraine-resistant lifestyle.

ADOPTION OF MIGRAINE DIET

Adopting a migraine-friendly diet can bring about several core benefits that contribute to managing and potentially alleviating the impact of migraines on one's life. Conversely, neglecting to adopt the right diet may lead to complications and exacerbate the frequency and severity of migraine episodes.

Core Benefits of Adopting a Migraine

Diet:

Trigger Identification and Reduction: A migraine diet involves identifying and avoiding specific trigger foods known to contribute to headaches. By understanding individual triggers and making informed dietary choices, individuals can significantly reduce the frequency and intensity of migraines

Stabilized Blood Sugar Levels: Consistent blood sugar levels are crucial for migraine prevention. The migraine diet emphasizes balanced meals and snacks, preventing the rapid spikes and crashes in blood sugar that can trigger headaches.

Nutrient-Rich Foods for Brain Health: The migraine diet focuses on nutrient-dense foods that support overall brain health. Incorporating fruits, vegetables, whole grains, and lean proteins provides essential vitamins and minerals that contribute to neurological well-being.

Hydration for Migraine Prevention: Proper hydration is a cornerstone of the migraine diet. Dehydration is a common trigger, and maintaining adequate fluid intake helps prevent headaches. Water, herbal teas, and other non-triggering beverages are encouraged.

Reduced Inflammation: Many migraine-friendly foods have anti-inflammatory properties. By emphasizing foods rich in antioxidants and omega-3 fatty acids, the migraine diet may contribute to reducing inflammation, which can be a factor in migraine development.

Improved Digestive Health: Some individuals experience gastrointestinal symptoms as part of their migraines. The migraine diet often includes foods that promote digestive health, contributing to overall well-being.

Complications of Not Adopting the Right

Migraine Diet:

Increased Migraine Frequency: If you don't follow a diet that reduces migraine triggers, you'll be exposed to possible triggers longer, which will increase the frequency of migraine attacks. One's everyday existence and general quality of life may be adversely affected by this.

Extended Recoveries: People may take longer to recover from migraine attacks if they don't follow a diet designed to avoid migraines. This may lead to longer bouts of pain and decreased functioning.

Dependency on drugs: People who are unable to control their migraines with diet may find themselves severely dependent on drugs. medicine overuse headaches and other adverse effects can result from over-reliance on medicine, which can further exacerbate the headache cycle.

Limited Lifestyle functioning: Daily activities and general functioning can be severely restricted by chronic migraines. People could be limited by the erratic character of their migraines if a migraine diet doesn't have a beneficial effect.

Diminished Overall Well-Being: The effects of migraines extend beyond the physical realm to include mental and emotional wellbeing. One factor that might lead to a decreased sense of wellbeing is not implementing a migraine diet that targets triggers and enhances general health.

In summary, implementing a diet tailored to migraineurs provides a comprehensive strategy for controlling migraines, resolving their causes, and enhancing general health. Ignoring to follow a proper diet can lead to many problems, which can affect migraine frequency and intensity as well as general quality of life. Making educated food decisions may be a potent weapon in the fight against migraines, giving sufferers a proactive and long-lasting method of controlling this neurological condition.

The Migraine Diet Recipes

Here are 10 migraine-friendly recipes with ingredients and instructions:

1. Quinoa and Vegetable Stir-Fry:

Ingredients:

- Quinoa
- Mixed vegetables (bell peppers, broccoli, carrots)
- Olive oil
- Garlic
- Low-sodium soy sauce

Instructions:

1. Cook quinoa according to package instructions.
2. In a pan, sauté garlic in olive oil.
3. Add mixed vegetables and stir-fry until tender.
4. Mix in cooked quinoa and soy sauce. Serve.

2. Salmon and Avocado Salad:

Ingredients:

- Salmon fillet
- Mixed greens
- Avocado
- Cherry tomatoes
- Lemon juice
- Olive oil

Instructions:

1. Grill or bake salmon until cooked.
2. Mix greens, diced avocado, and halved cherry tomatoes in a bowl.
3. Top with flaked salmon.
4. Drizzle with a dressing made of lemon juice and olive oil.

3. Turkey and Veggie Lettuce Wraps:

Ingredients:

- Ground turkey

- Lettuce leaves
- Bell peppers
- Onion
- Cumin, paprika, salt, and pepper

Instructions:

1. Sauté ground turkey with diced onion and bell peppers.
2. Season with cumin, paprika, salt, and pepper.
3. Spoon the turkey mixture onto lettuce leaves to create wraps.

4. Sweet Potato and Chickpea Curry:

Ingredients:

- Sweet potatoes
- Chickpeas
- Coconut milk
- Curry powder
- Onion
- Garlic

Instructions:

1. Sauté chopped onion and garlic in a pot.
2. Add diced sweet potatoes, chickpeas, coconut milk, and curry powder.
3. Simmer until sweet potatoes are tender.

5. Greek Yogurt Parfait:

Ingredients:

- Greek yogurt
- Berries (blueberries, strawberries)
- Honey
- Almonds (optional)

Instructions:

1. Layer Greek yogurt with fresh berries in a glass.
2. Drizzle with honey and top with almonds if desired.

6. Egg and Spinach Omelette:

Ingredients:

- Eggs
- Spinach
- Cherry tomatoes
- Feta cheese (optional)

Instructions:

1. Whisk eggs and pour into a heated pan.
2. Add spinach, halved cherry tomatoes, and feta.
3. Cook until eggs are set, then fold in half.

7. Cucumber and Hummus Sandwich:

Ingredients:

- Whole grain bread
- Cucumber
- Hummus
- Turkey slices (optional)

Instructions:

1. Spread hummus on whole grain bread.
2. Layer with cucumber slices and turkey if desired.

8. Brown Rice and Vegetable Bowl:

Ingredients:

- Brown rice
- Broccoli
- Carrots
- Edamame
- Teriyaki sauce

Instructions:

1. Cook brown rice and steam vegetables.
2. Toss with teriyaki sauce and serve.

9. Banana and Almond Smoothie:

Ingredients:

- Banana

- Almond milk
- Almond butter
- Ice cubes

Instructions:

Blend banana, almond milk, almond butter, and ice cubes until smooth.

10. Mango and Coconut Chia Pudding:

Ingredients:

- Chia seeds
- Coconut milk
- Mango
- Honey

Instructions:

1. Mix chia seeds with coconut milk and refrigerate until thick.
2. Layer with diced mango and drizzle with honey.

These recipes are designed to incorporate nutrient-dense, migraine-friendly ingredients while offering a variety of flavors to suit different preferences.

Building A Migraine-Friendly Plate

Building a migraine-friendly plate is a fundamental aspect of adopting a dietary approach to manage and potentially alleviate migraine symptoms. The goal is to create balanced meals that contribute to stable blood sugar levels, minimize potential triggers, and provide essential nutrients for overall well-being.

1. Emphasize Whole Foods:

Start by focusing on whole, unprocessed foods. Incorporate a variety of fruits, vegetables, lean proteins, whole grains, and healthy fats into your meals. Whole foods provide a rich array of vitamins, minerals, and antioxidants that support neurological health.

2. Balance Macronutrients:

Aim for a balanced distribution of macronutrients –
carbohydrates, proteins, and fats – in each meal.
This balance helps maintain steady blood sugar
levels, reducing the risk of headaches triggered by
rapid fluctuations in glucose.

3. Watch Portion Sizes:

Pay attention to portion sizes to avoid overeating,
which can contribute to digestive discomfort and
potentially trigger migraines. Eating smaller, more
frequent meals throughout the day can help stabilize
energy levels and prevent blood sugar spikes.

4. Identify Trigger Foods:

Keep a migraine diary to identify specific trigger
foods that may contribute to headaches. Common
triggers include certain cheeses, processed meats,
chocolate, and foods containing artificial additives.
Once identified, minimize or eliminate these
triggers from your plate.

5. Stay Hydrated:

Dehydration is a known migraine trigger, so prioritize adequate fluid intake. Water is the best choice, but herbal teas and diluted fruit juices can also contribute to hydration.

6. Mindful Eating:

Practice mindful eating by paying attention to hunger and fullness cues. Eat in a calm environment, savoring each bite without distractions. This approach can help prevent overeating and reduce stress, a potential migraine trigger.

7. Limit Caffeine and Alcohol:

While moderate amounts of caffeine may have some benefits, excessive intake can trigger migraines. Similarly, alcohol can be a trigger for some individuals. Moderation and awareness of personal tolerance levels are key.

8. Customize for Individual Needs:

Recognize that everyone's triggers and dietary needs are unique. Experiment with different foods and observe their impact on your migraines. Consider consulting with a healthcare professional or a registered dietitian to tailor your diet to your specific requirements.

Building a migraine-friendly plate is about creating a sustainable and enjoyable approach to eating that aligns with your health goals. By adopting a balanced and personalized dietary strategy, individuals can take proactive steps to manage migraines and enhance their overall well-being.

Conclusion

In summary, following a diet that is migraine-friendly becomes clear as a comprehensive approach to general wellbeing as well as a method for controlling migraines. Beyond only lessening the frequency and severity of headaches, this dietary change has other positive effects on one's overall health and way of life.

Through careful meal planning that emphasizes full, nutrient-dense foods, people can achieve blood sugar stabilization, decreased inflammation, and enhanced cognitive function. By fostering a relationship between the person and their food, eating habits that incorporate mindfulness can lead to a mindful and fulfilling meal experience.

Using a migraine journal to identify and eliminate trigger foods gives people back control over their health. Because each person's triggers are unique, this individualized approach helps people feel empowered and in control of their migraine management.

Adopting a diet that is conducive to migraines goes beyond reactive management. It takes a proactive approach, focusing on prevention via smart dietary decisions and lifestyle modifications. Whether it's maintaining hydration, adjusting the diet to meet specific demands, or balancing macronutrients, this method turns eating habits into a weapon for resilience against migraine episodes.

When people see improvements in their health, such as greater energy and less need for medicine, adopting a migraine-friendly diet becomes more than just a routine—it becomes a sustainable way of life. This is not a voyage of deprivation, but an exploration of the bounty of tasty, nutrient-dense meals that fuel the body and the mind.

Essentially, following a diet that is migraine-friendly is an expression of a desire to live a life that is less controlled by migraines and more full of energy, equilibrium, and long-term health. It is an effective and widely available way to take back control of one's health, enabling people to enjoy life's special moments without having to live in constant pain.

Contact Us

Dear Reader,

If you have any questions, need further clarification, or require assistance with any aspect of the book, please do not hesitate to reach out to me. I am more than happy to provide additional insights, address your queries, or simply engage in a meaningful discussion.

Feel free to contact me at: IsabelleHartleyBooks@gmail.com. Your feedback and inquiries are always welcome.

FREE 30 DAYS MEAL PLANNER

FREE 30Days Meal Planner, a priceless extra to get you started on the path to a more organized and healthy living. This meticulously curated planner is made to make meal planning easier, save you time, and help you meet your nutritional objectives. Prepare to enjoy the advantages of this wonderful resource! Scan the QR Code below now.